Disclaimer

TABLE OF CONTENTS

Contents

Introduction

This workbook is a tool for managing nutrition.   Losing body fat is based 5% on education, 80% on food, and 15% of exercise and movement. Diet plays the largest role in weight loss and fitness.

Education + Nutrition + Optimal Movement (exercise,daily activity) = Total Fitness

Many variables impact nutrition management.   There are behaviors, as well as physical challenges involved in managing food. Nutrition is complicated and requires understanding, effort, and patience.

This workbook divides into four (4) modules due to the difficulty associated with nutrition management. You will complete 1 module per week for four weeks. Skills in this workbook are broken down into manageable activities that allow for discovery, understanding, and learning.

Module	Description
1 (Week 1)	Setting Goals, objectives
2 (Week 2)	measurements Logging and Monitoring
3 (Week 3)	Understanding Physical and Behavior Hunger
4 (Week 4)	Establishing support

Where possible, this workbook works best in conjunction with a professionally certified personal trainer & sports nutritionist who can provide counseling and evaluation. A professional trainer brings experience and knowledge that can reduce time and effort in reaching your goals.

Everyone has lapses in managing hunger and appetite suppression. The issue is not whether you will fail, but how you will deal with failure. Everyone fails at nutrition while trying to lose weight and become fit. Strategy for Fitness™ helps you develop a vision of success. It provides a road map for attaining the vision while contributing to understanding the skills and behaviors necessary to provide sustained weight loss and total fitness.

Along with this workbook, there are reference materials in the form of articles, internet links, and forms. You need to take advantage of these recommendations to enhance your knowledge about nutrition management.

Managing diet requires making lifestyle changes. As your skills and behaviors develop, fitness becomes easier. You are encouraged to optimize a strategy for fitness to facilitate change and improve your expertise and practices which will lead to a healthy and fit body. Workouts and meal programs, along with logging systems are readily available via the internet. The internet also provides a gold mind of nutritional videos, podcasts, and blogs that will prove useful in reaching your goals. This workbook will help you organize the information you gather in a way that will optimize what is learned to help you achieve your fitness goals. This book will also assist in determining what to look for on the internet and what products will work best towards attaining your goals

When you have clearly articulated a vision, the next step is to compare it to your current reality. Measurements can help paint a clear picture of your need for change. The biggest barrier you have is denying your current fitness and health status. Information is power. It provides the means to govern and manage your destiny. You have the ability, with accurate information, to develop clear plans and actions to achieve your vision. Honest and reliable information also allows you to establish your plan within a realistic period. Many people fail to implement fitness programs because they expect too much too quickly. People often quit because they cannot achieve immediate weight loss. Accurately comparing your current fitness level with your desired level gives a good indication of changes needed, and how long it will take to achieve your fitness goals.

Do not rely on one measurement. Your vision will contain more than one result. Some of the results are physical measurements, e.g. dropping three waist sizes, yet others will be behavior measures, e.g. people complimenting you on how good you look. It is important to define benchmarks that will help you see progress, as well as indicate when you have achieved your vision. Some mileposts are better suited for long-term trend analysis such as the weight scale. Others are more suited to short-term analysis, e.g. body fat percentage and body circumference. Make sure you define measures that are acceptable to achieving your goals.

Module 1

Setting Goals, Objectives, and Measurements

Defining the future is your first task. Establish a clear vision of your future fitness. Having a plan is the best way to reduce uncertainty about reaching your fitness goal. Your investment of time and money should produce a tangible result. Begin by creating your vision.

A vision definition needs to be concrete. Concrete means measurements must be tangible, viewable, and data based. Start by defining how your body will look and feel when you have reached your goal, e.g. shape, size, contours, endurance, flexibility, and strength. Athletes use this approach to visualize a basketball shot or a particular ice skating move. The brain has the power to imagine a future state and move the body towards that state.

We are creatures of habit. Over time, we learn habits through repetition. Behavior changes the same way. Learning through behavior change and repetition means you can create new habits that are good for fitness and reinforce those habits through repetition.

If change is desirable but doesn't happen, you didn't want change. The desire to change has to outweigh the desire to remain the same.

People create various excuses to resist change, e.g. time, money, or physical limitations. Time is dependent on prioritizing. When your health and wellness becomes critical, you will prioritize the time to eat right and workout. Why wait until it 's hard? Below is a tool that can help you create a vision:

VISION TOOL

"You are speaking in front of a large audience on the topic of your successful fitness transformation. You have 5 minutes to express your feelings about achieving your vision and how it has changed your life."

Answer: Write your answer to the above question below. Try to use definable measures, e.g. clothes sizes, more energy, etc. Paint a picture your audience can visualize.

Flesh out some specifics of your vision, i.e. I have lost 80 lbs of fat, dropped from 38% to 22% body fat, and lost 25 inches in body circumference. I am not as tired. I went from a size 48 jeans to 36. I am getting compliments about my appearance every day. Some people have visions other than weight loss, e.g. improved blood sugar, lower triglycerides, or more stamina.

The concept establishes critical measurements that determine your final success and your progress along the way. Measurements are necessary for setting goals and determining realistic time spans. They assess progress and help keep you focused. Without measurements, the path to success can be fraught with uncertainty and trouble. Measures stabilize you during your change process.

Seek out a professional trainer to help you establish your measurements. There are several tools available for tracking and monitoring measures. The core tests are below:

- Body circumference, e.g. inches around the arms, waist, stomach, hip, thighs, calves, and neck. Some trainers include the chest.
- Body fat %
- Weight (Primarily a long term trend measurement)
- Physical fitness, e.g. strength, endurance, flexibility, etc.

Use several different measurements to determine success as opposed to using one, e.g. weight. For example, if a person lost two pounds of fat and gained one pound of muscle, their scale weight would show zero loss or gain. Neutral weight loss in this circumstance happens because muscle weighs more than fat. When gaining muscle, the body loses inches. Muscle molecules are more compressed and denser than fat molecules. They take up less space on the body. Also, the body has to burn more calories to sustain one pound of muscle, versus one pound of fat. Gaining muscle is a desirable outcome of fitness, which the weight scale did not indicate. Using several measurements consistently is the best approach for making progress towards fitness.

At this point, stop and go to the analysis page, complete the starting measurements, and establish some goals with time parameters. You will track these objectives on a regular basis to help determine your progress. As you measure, record the information, and define your development. Measurements will indicate any changes you need to make in your strategy.

Other measurements are personal in nature. These are behavioral measures. On your nutritional monitoring, there are applications you can place on your SmartPhones and tablets like MyFitnessPal; these apps provide a place to log your measurements, and thoughts. Keeping a journal will help reinforce those less easily measured aspects of your goals, for example how you feel about yourself at a particular time, if others are recognizing your change, and if you are engaging in more activities like dancing, or playing with the kids. Make sure you start your journal immediately. Your first journal entries normally are fears and skepticisms. As you progress, you should feel a definite positive change in your entries. A journal is a powerful tool linking your fitness and nutrition activities to your outcomes through measurements. One client was able to tie his HDL and LDL reversal to his aerobic and resistance exercises through his journal entries. As he recorded his aerobic activity and his blood test results over time, he noticed improvement correlations between exercise and increased HDL cholesterol. His journal provided a history that apparently linked cholesterol change to his activity and made him feel better about exercising. At this point, go to MyFitnessPal and start recording in your journal.

Next, you should start monitoring your nutritional intake. Watching your calories requires an understanding of two basic nutritional concepts. The first concept is how calories affect your fitness. Secondly, you need to know about your metabolism.

Module 2

Logging and Monitoring

Control begins by understanding your needs and how they relate to your vision and goals. You need to determine exactly how many calories to consume and burn each day, in order reach your desired fitness level.

Understanding Calories and the metabolism

The saying, "A calorie is a calorie is a calorie" has a grain of truth to it, but it is not the whole story. Calories are important when setting goals for weight loss or gain. However, calories are not all created equal. There are differences in fat calories, e.g. fish oils are healthier than hydrogenated oils. Fibrous carbohydrates are better for you than simple carbs. With protein, there are differences between animal protein vs. plant protein.

To grasp how calories affect the body, a brief explanation of metabolism will prove helpful. There are two hormones released as part of the metabolic function. One is insulin the other is glucagon. Insulin is released to cope with excess sugar and fats placed in the blood stream not processed by the liver. Insulin inhibits fat burning when released. Glucagon processes food (calories) into fuel that creates energy. Glucagon increases fat burning. The key is to keep these two hormones balanced. When these hormones are balanced, the body both loses weight and builds lean muscle mass.

Nutrition is the key to managing insulin and glucagon. To manage food, you must know how different carbohydrates, fats, and proteins affect these hormones. Defining your metabolic type is the first step to understanding how your body turns carbohydrates, fats, and proteins into calories. To find your metabolic type go to www.naturallyhealthyyellowpages.com.
Complete the metabolic survey, score the survey, and download the data from your results. This site provides a brief explanation of each metabolic type. The data from this site will help you establish a nutritional plan. You can also, find a basic description of metabolic types listed in Isabel Del Los Rios's book *The Diet Solution* found at www.thedietsolutionprogram.com a highly recommended reading.

Based on your goals, either consume fewer calories than you burn to lose weight or consume more calories than you burn to gain weight. It is just a little more complicated than consuming fewer or more calories; it is also important to gain muscle mass while losing, or gaining weight. Muscle provides you the strength and energy to accomplish your daily activities. Your caloric need is based on your body type, age, weight, and lifestyle. Below is the formula for determining your calorie needs.

Survival Calories

The first step in establishing a solid nutritional program is determining the number of calories needed for a given day. You begin by determining your Basal Metabolic Rate (BMR), the number of calories your body needs to survive if you did nothing but lie on your bed for twenty-four hours. BMR takes into account your basic body functions like breathing and digestion. The best-known approach to determining your BMR is the formula below:

Harris-Benedict formula for Basal Metabolic Rate (BMR)

(The calories you burn just to sustain your body's life)

Women:

BMR = 655 + (4.35 x weight in pounds) + (4.7 x height in inches) - (4.7 x age in years)

Example:

A Woman 5' 8" tall, weighing 150 pounds and is forty years old: 655 + (4.35 X 150 pounds) + (4.7 X 68 inches) – (4.7 X 40) =1439 calories per day

Men: BMR = 66 + (6.23 x weight in pounds) + (12.7 x height in inches) -
(6.8 x age in year)

The above shows our female example needs 1439 calories per day just to maintain life. It does not take into account any other activities. The Harris-Benedict formula is currently one of the best ways to determine your BMR, given no formula can account for all issues of the body. Make sure you pay attention to the difference between the men's and women's formula.

Lifestyle Calories

The next step after determining your BMR is to identify your lifestyle trend. Lifestyles identify the additional calories needed to sustain your energy throughout the day. Lifestyles are sedated, active, moderately active, and very active. Taking extreme examples, a person who is a customer call representative and sits at a computer all day then goes home and watches television would have a sedated lifestyle.

On the other end of the scale is the very active lifestyle. An example of this would be the bricklayer who worked all day mixing cement, carrying bricks, laying bricks, and digging ditches, then mowed the lawn.

It does not take much to realize, if they both ate about 1800 calories a day, given the same age, height, and weight, the sedated person would start to gain weight because he/she burned far fewer calories. Conversely, the very active person might feel tired and worn down because they didn't consume enough calories to meet their lifestyle need. The average person burns an additional 600 calories during their waking hours, assuming an active person with no exercise routines. You can determine your daily caloric need by using an activity multiplier like the one below:

Activity Multiplier

Sedentary =   BMR X 1.20 (little or no exercise, desk job)
Lightly active =   BMR X 1.375 (light exercise/sports 1-3 days/wk)
Moderately active =   BMR X 1.55 (moderate exercise/sports 3-5 days/wk)
Very active =   BMR X 1.725 (hard exercise/sports 6-7 days/wk)
Extra active =   BMR X 1.90 (hard daily exercise/sports & physical job)

Her BMR is 1439 calories per day, rounded.
Her activity level is sedentary (little or no exercise, desk job) 1.20
Her total daily energy expenditure in calories = 1.20 X 1439 = **1727**

calories/day

At this point, you should plug in your numbers to determine your calorie needs. Your trainer can help you develop your calorie needs based on your workout program, and lifestyle. Also, your coach regularly provides a targeted heart rate that will help guide your exercise program.

One pound of fat equals 3500 calories. If your desire is to lose weight safely, you will average two pounds of fat per week. Losing two pounds of fat per week requires burning 7000 calories less than you consume each week. Keep in mind that different calories, e.g. fat, carbohydrates, and proteins affect your metabolism differently. These calorie variances affect your ability to process them efficiently. To lose two pounds per week, divide 7000 calories by 7, and subtract this from your daily calorie needs, developed previously. The new number is your new daily calorie requirements adjusted for two pounds of fat loss. Make sure all your daily requirements are added in before subtracting the calories for weight loss. This calculation ensures you have enough calories to meet all your daily needs. When you exercise, adjust your daily calories for exercise days to ensure you have enough energy to workout.

Now that you know your metabolic type, you need to select foods that balance insulin and glucagon in a way that optimizes fat burning while building muscle. Balancing, insulin, and glucagon require choosing the right foods to fit your metabolic type. You can use the internet to find websites that can provide foods based on metabolic type. For you to stick with the program, you need to choose the right foods that you will like.

As you lose weight, you will adjust your calorie need over time. The less you weigh, the fewer calories you need. You will have different calorie needs on days when you exercise, e.g. weight training. Logging your food intake on **MyFitnessPal** will provide the proper breakdown of calories eaten. From this information, you can adjust your foods to meet your metabolic type.

Monitoring Tools

Many software programs help you monitor calories by carbohydrates, fats, and protein consumption. Some software tools can help you create grocery lists. These are very useful nutrition management tools when combined with journals. They provide calendars, goal setting, food charts, and apps for your Iphone™ or PDA. They help you track your information quickly no matter where you go. One such program on the internet is MyFitnessPal.com. Go to this site and establish your account. In the beginning, you need to monitor your food consumption and activities daily. Upgrading is worth the investment to have these programs available for monitoring and tracking. They will save you lots of time, and provide a more accurate assessment of your calorie intake, and burn. People, who record calorie intake from memory, often underestimate food calories by as much as thirty percent.

It is time to create your calorie need and establish a monitoring and logging process. Take some time right now to become very familiar with MyFitnessPal. Learn how to use all the tools on this valuable app to manage your fitness progress.

Module 3

Understanding Physical & Behavioral Hunger

Since 80% of your success is nutrition, it makes sense to know what factors drive your hunger. Have you ever found yourself walking by a restaurant and smelling steak on the grill? Did your mouth start watering and your stomach start churning? You were captive to a food trigger. Somewhere in your life, you associated the smell of a grilling steak with satisfying your hunger. Food triggers begin early in life, as a child, and gets stronger the more you reinforce the behavior. You think this is physically driven hunger because you feel hungry, but it it is a behaviorally driven desire. You need to understand the difference between what your body needs (physical hunger), and what is a desire (behavioral hunger).

Physical Hunger

Your body requires the intake of food and liquids to survive. It is a miracle and produces many of the enzymes, amino acids, and nutrients it needs. It requires food and liquids to provide additional nutrients, enzymes, and amino acids it does not produce. Consequently, your body sends you signals based on several factors to eat and drink. Hunger signals happen about every 3-4 hours. Hunger happens about the time it takes the body to digest and process your last meal. You can deduce from this, how you came to eat three meals a day. If you eat smaller and healthier meals, you will usually satisfy your hunger. When you eat three meals, versus six to eight meals a day, you will eat more calories. Eating three meals a day can quickly overcome the physical hunger problem. If you track how many times you eat, typically you will eat more than three times a day. Most people are snacking in between larger meals all day long.

Snacking is often driven by behavioral hunger. The dilemma is, you are not in control of your eating. Habitual eating places you out of control. Why not put yourself in control? Research has shown the body metabolizes food better when eating six to eight small meals a day versus three larger meals. When eating smaller meals, there is less desire to eat large amounts of sugar, salt, and fat at one time. Your body's metabolism has to work harder to burn the calories you are consuming.

If you eat the right foods for your metabolic type, you will reduce cravings. Eating the right foods combined with frequent eating will control your hunger. You will have to remind yourself to snack at the proper time because your body will not be sending a hunger signal from the brain. You read this right! You should eat more frequently. When you eat smaller amounts regularly, you eat fewer calories per meal. Eating more often reduces hunger. Your body also processes food more efficiently, because it is processing fewer calories per meal.

It takes discipline and planning to eat properly. The biggest problem is deciding what snacks to eat during the morning and afternoon. Eat meals that follow the guidelines associated with your metabolic type, i.e. if you are a protein type you will want to ensure your snack has protein in it, and combine it with the right carbohydrate. Prepare and package your snacks and meals in advance. Preparation will help you during busy days, and while you travel. As a society, we are mobile and have more family members working. It is harder to manage snacks and meals out than it is to prepare them at home. Food quality and timing is where planning becomes necessary.

The food and snack industry has one mission, for you to eat more combinations of fat, sugar, and salt. This combination is addictive and creates the desire to eat more. Food companies spend millions of dollars on research to get you to eat more food. It is no different from what the tobacco industry has done to addict smokers. The big difference is, you do not have to smoke, but you have to eat. You must eat to survive. The food industry's objective is profit, not your health. The food industry has become sensitive to the health craze. They are designing products and advertising that aligns with today's health fad. The problem is, their ads are deceptive, if not downright lies. They maneuver labeling on their packages to emphasize health, taking advantage of the uneducated, i.e., food packaged as low fat often has additional sugar. It is your responsibility to educate yourself about labeling and ingredients.

You have to decide what foods to eat, and when to eat them. Knowing what foods are healthy is critical to your success. Take the time to research about fats, carbohydrates, and proteins, and then decide what foods are best for each of these nutrients. Pay less attention to advertising and more attention to research. Become educated so you can make sensible food choices. Place yourself in control of nutrition instead of the food industries. You can find out more about fats, carbohydrates, and proteins by reading Building a Strategy For Fitness: a model to reach and sustain total fitness & health by Vic Vogel the companion book for this workbook.

You need to establish a schedule for eating. You have to be jealous about your eating plan. Make a commitment to prioritize your health, and assign enough time to achieve your priority.

Being persistent means not letting other things get in the way of your eating plan. You have to set alarms and traps to help you remember to eat at the right times. Eating
the right food at the right time is critical to building a fit and healthy body.

You should shop for food and snacks that are portable, tasty, easy to eat, natural, and not prepackaged, e.g. apples. Identify foods and drinks that fit your needs, which you will like, and still fall within healthy eating guidelines.

To curb physical hunger simply eat 6-8 small meals a day. You should stay within your calorie goals, and minimize the amount of simple and complex carbohydrates. Consume fewer carbs during late afternoon and evening. Your meals should consist of the right balance of carbohydrates, proteins, and fats. This combination of quality food and frequent eating will satisfy your physical hunger cravings, and provide necessary nutrients.

Also, it is important to consume approximately 64 ounces of water a day. A tip to help you curb overeating at lunch and dinner is to drink at least 8 ounces of water 30 minutes before eating lunch, or dinner. Drinking water prior your meal will curb your physical appetite. In many cases, the physical craving can appear to be food oriented, but often the craving is dehydration. When you have a physical need for food outside your normal eating schedule, you should drink some water, wait twenty minutes, then see if you are still hungry before eating. Drink water when drinking alcohol.

Behavioral Hunger

Often hunger is triggered by something other than physical hunger. We find ourselves eating out of habit, or reacting to something smelling good. These are behavioral cues, which are not associated with our body's need to take in food for energy. The danger of this eating pattern is exceeding our required calorie intake. Most of the time it is more carbohydrates, versus protein or fat that we crave. The body does not feel the need for food and thus ends up storing it as fat for later use. Today there is less need for fat to jumpstart our body. Thus, fat keeps accumulating, resulting in obesity.

Behavioral hunger is harder to conquer than physical hunger. Habits or emotional desires drive behavioral eating. Behavioral eating correlates with pleasing or relieving such behaviors as stress. Since these are self-induced behaviors, it requires you to change your thought processes to overcome the hunger pains.

With today's television marketing, you are vulnerable to food driven advertising campaigns. These attacks focus on triggering your thoughts about food products like fries. Consequently, your brain creates a sensation of smelling and tasting French fries. The association between smell and pleasure within your brain drives you to eat more French fries. It is important to recognize you have these thoughts and learn to identify them and disrupt them.

First, you have to challenge the ideas. Once you recognize you are craving chips, and a burger, use a phrase like, "I am not hungry right now." You can also challenge the thought, by thinking about how much exercise you will have to do to burn off the calories, i.e." I will have to walk 45 additional minutes to burn off the 300 calories in that small order of
Chips and a hamburger."

Secondly, substitute a different pleasurable thought. Think about how rejecting fries has helped tighten up your belt two more notches to a size 36 jeans instead of size 38. Reward yourself mentally for overcoming your thought by placing a star on the calendar of the refrigerator. Journaling helps to track your thoughts and proves useful in making
needed changes to behavior.

Thirdly, change your circumstances. For example, when you anticipate commercials mute the television and do something. Put clothes up from the laundry, or read more about proper nutrition, then return to the program. Exercising during commercials not only takes your mind off eating but also has health benefits.

You will find yourself making mistakes or cheating. Cheating is normal. Everybody does it. What you need to understand is the difference between a mere lapse, and returning to your original problem. The key is to realize the problem. If it is a lapse, you can overcome it by identifying it as a failure and returning to strategies you used previously. In the end, you will still achieve your goal. If you falter and find yourself giving into a craving and you associate that with failure, you may decide to scrub the whole program as hopeless. It is important to allow yourself an item you crave in restricted quantity, to help overcome the desire to have it.

Having a cookie periodically will not destroy your whole program, as long as you are in control of the type and size of the cookie. You should not do this until you have mastered entirely resisting the cookie. If you cannot, then you have to say no to the cookie. Any attempt to rationalize will lead to increasing consumption of cookies.

You manage cravings through portion control or committing to additional exercise activity. If you become too strict about your program, it will not be appealing to you, and you will not adhere to your plan. As you stick with the plan, it becomes easier, and you can improve the plan in small increments over time. After all, you do have your whole life to make this work.

Monitor and track your thoughts throughout the week. In the reference section is a form to help identify your feelings about cravings. Use this form to help you recognize desires and to overcome them through alternative strategies.

Most behavioral eating patterns align with time, activities, places, smells, or emotional issues. To change your behavior, you must identify the behavior that is causing the problem. Once this is completed, you need to determine a strategy for changing the behavior. You have to believe change is necessary to you. Without the felt need to change, no program will force you to make the change, at least on a sustained basis. You need to define your problem. Identifying and designing strategies to overcome your eating behaviors is liberating. It will change your body into a healthy and fit body. You will receive compliments and improve your self-esteem. Overcoming setbacks strengthens your ability to sustain fitness. Overcoming obstacles will is covered in an upcoming module about support. Now is the time for you to identify the hunger cravings you have, and categorize them as physical or behavioral. Use the form in the reference section to log your physical and behavioral hunger cravings. Once you complete this task write down strategies that will help you overcome them.

During this week, develop strategies to overcome your cravings. Establish a schedule for eating, and what foods to eat. Scheduling starts your process of change. It requires sustaining your change process as events affect your life. You should always keep the alarms and traps you established, in place as reminders for controlling your hunger. In the end, the accountability for change will be solely on your shoulders. Only you can decide to control your behavioral hunger.

Your objective this week is to identify your physical and behavioral hunger. Next, develop strategies to overcome them. Make notes in your journal about how well you have done, or problems you are having. Log your craving and thoughts as they occur, and develop strategies to overcome them. Your trainer/nutritionist will set aside time during your sessions to cover how you are progressing. Occasionally a full training period will be required to help overcome these issues. Remember nutrition is as important, if not more important than the physical training. Think about the time you spend on food control as an investment in your life.

Module 4

Establishing Support

A professional trainer will be your best support source. He/She will give you access to information quickly. A personal trainer is going to provide honest feedback. Other support sources can be less accurate, and in many cases encourage bad fitness habits. Your trainer provides you essential information on nutrition, exercise form, and most importantly safety. Frequently uninformed people start training programs that can injure them, leading them to stop using the program. Investing in a trainer is a smart decision.

In addition to your coach, you need a support team that will help you attain your goals. During your journey towards total fitness, there will be many personal barriers you will have to overcome, e.g. eating habits, stress, and time. There are also external barriers that can influence your ability to become fit, e.g. work, family, and school.

You don't live in an isolated environment. Your environment affects your eating habits. If you are in business, you may have to attend a business dinner. There will be social events for the family. Particularly stressful situations are Thanksgiving, Christmas, birthdays, marriages, and showers. In America, we have established the tradition of serving food at these occasions. When attending these events, not eating gets you chastised for not being part of the family or team.

Addressing these issues is no small feat. In addition to social events, you have to deal with those that are close to you, e.g. spouse, brother, sister, mother, father, or boyfriend. Behaviors range from excitement to jealousy. Fitness programs cause disruptive relationships between partners.

Jealousy occurs as one spouse makes progress and the other does not. In some families, being obese has been part of the tradition. If you decide to become fit, you challenge the family's history, leading to comments like, "There are a lot of us who are heavy, and we have done just beautiful." These observations are meant to maintain the status quo. These can be serious issues if not addressed early in your decision to improve your fitness.

There are external barriers you will have to address, e.g. your friends, work associates, and church members. Many of these people see you regularly and will become aware of your changes. Beware of the subtle comments like, "Oh, I notice you have lost some weight, how fantastic." Jealousy is also prevalent in the workplace. You will be achieving goals that others want, but have not made the commitment to undertake. On the other hand, you will find lots of support from people who wonder what you are doing to achieve your progress. It is rewarding to serve as a witness to others.

Other barriers are not people oriented. Those professionals dedicated to their careers, find themselves using time as an excuse. Time is an easy excuse to develop. People are quick to blame something else, e.g. work for their lack of discipline. You will have to identify these issues upfront and develop strategies to overcome these concerns.

All these barriers seem insurmountable. It is not as bad as it sounds. The trick is to get support, and not let the obstacles manage you. You plan daily, whether it is your workload, shopping, kids, or family events. You can do the same for your health and wellness. When your health and wellness

deteriorates, the rest of your world suffers, including you. If you don't manage your fitness, you will be too tired to be with your family and friends. Your work will suffer. Illness will become more frequent in your life. The list of negative impacts can be endless. The most important

priority you have is YOU! Without your health, you are less than you can be for yourself, your family, and your work. Decide right now that you cannot do this alone. You will need support from a host of other people. Once you cross this threshold, you will find it much easier to achieve your fitness goal. Not only will you hit your goals, but you will also exceed your expectations sooner.

So what is the first thing you need to do? The first thing is to make a list of potential barriers. Listing barriers seem silly, but writing them down, and assessing the barriers will save you time and headaches. In the reference section is a form to help you list the obstacles that might prevent you from achieving your goals. **TAKE THE TIME TO FILL IT OUT NOW!**

First, list your barrier. Next, identify the source(s) of your barrier. Then prioritize the barrier's importance and difficulty. In the comments section, list ways you might prevent the barrier from happening.

Another tool to help gain support from family, friends, co-workers and associates is a contract between you, and them. The first step is to list the people you feel will provide active support. Next, list the people who might be enablers or negative influences. After registering these people generate a contract (a sample contract appears in the reference section). Read the contract to them. You could have individual meetings with some people. For others, a group session may be more appropriate. Make sure they understand the fine points of the contract and their role in

supporting you. Have each person sign the contract. Let them know you appreciate their help. It is important to keep your supporters informed about your progress so they can share in your success.

Below are some hints for overcoming barriers. You should add to them, and use this exercise to help you become aware of the issues you will need to manage. Again, you can ask for help from your trainer/nutritionist, or refer to websites for information to help.

Hints:

1. Make a list of barriers, and prioritize them based on; the likelihood of the obstacles is happening, and their difficulty to overcome if they do happen.

2. Make a list of everyone you know that will be around you, and categorize them as supporters or enablers. Develop a support contract, and get them to sign the contract with you.

3. Thank those who support you.

4. Use grace and kindness when reminding others of their enabling habits.
5. Share your excitement about your progress with your supporters.

6. Attack your most challenging and highest priority barriers first. Take them on one at a time, i.e. "I am going to turn off the TV and get up and do something active all this week." Then move on to the next barrier.

7. Do not go overboard. There will be things you cannot control. It is important to recognize when you have given into a wall and make an effort to correct it as soon as possible.

8. Remove all food obstacles from your house. Clean out your Kitchen, and office space. Stock your kitchen with foods that align with your metabolic meal plan.

9. If you can't resist the vending machine, find someplace else to take your break. Go for a walk.

10. Continually educate yourself about how certain foods affect you. Knowledge is one of the strongest resources for overcoming barriers.

11. Stay in touch with your trainer/nutritionist. Log what you eat, and when you eat.

12. Write in your journal when you are having trouble, or experiencing success, and send it to your trainer/nutritionist. Compare your activities and eating with your journal notes.

Best wishes on your journey to total fitness and health.

Victor

RESOURCES

Monitoring Hunger Thoughts

What was your thought, e.g. I am craving a candy bar.	Strategy: What did you do to overcome your thoughts, e.g. Resisted by thinking how much more time I would have to run to neutralize the calories from the candy bar.	Results: Decided against the candy bar and chose a small packet of salt free nuts to curb my appetite.	Time of Day: 19:20 AM

PHYSICAL / HUNGER BEHAVIOR

PHYSICAL CHARACTERISTICS	PHYSICAL APPETITE	BEHAVIORAL APPETITE
Physical symptoms	Stomach pangs, lightheaded, dizzy	none
Desires	Desire to eat something, not a specific craving	A specific craving, e.g. wanting a donut after walking by a donut shop.
Appetite Phase	3-5 hours after last meal	Environmental factors e.g. times, places, smells, behavioral stress
Control	Eat frequent small meals during the day	Change environment, e.g. do not walk by donut shop, fight triggers by replacing triggers with opposing thoughts.

Body Cirrcumfernce Measurement Chart

Measurement	Start
Resting Heart Rate	
Neck	
Right Arm	
Left Arm	
2" (5cm) Above Navel	
Navel	
2" (5cm) Below Navel	
Hips	
Right thigh	
Left Thigh	
Right Calf	
Left Calf	
Total Body Inches	

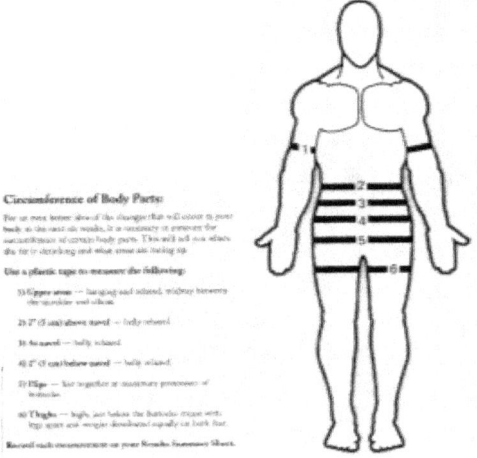

Circumference of Body Parts:

For an even better idea of the changes that will occur to your body in the next six weeks, it is necessary to measure the circumference of certain body parts. This will tell you where the fat is shrinking and what areas are firming up.

Use a plastic tape to measure the following:

1) Upper arm — hanging and relaxed, midway between the shoulder and elbow.

2) 2" (5 cm) above navel — belly relaxed.

3) At navel — belly relaxed.

4) 2" (5 cm) below navel — belly relaxed.

5) Hips — feet together at maximum protrusion of buttocks.

6) Thighs — high, just below the buttocks crease with legs apart and weight distributed equally on both feet.

Record each measurement on your Results Statement Sheet.

Measure each part of the body in the same place each time you measure.

Body Measurement Chart

Measurement	Start	1st Remeasure
	2/25/11	3/18/11
Right Arm	13.75	14.25
Left Arm	13	13.5
2" (5cm) Above Navel	45.25	44
Navel	48	48
2" (5cm) Below Navel	53.5	52.5
Hips	57.5	55.5
Right thigh	33.5	30
Left Thigh	32.5	27.5
Right Calf	17	17
Left Calf	18	18
Neck	14.25	
		13.75
Total Body Inches		
Resting Heart Rate	59	
	47	
Age		
Percent Body Fat	37.90%	35%
	245	239
Weight		
	172	
Lean Muscle Mass		
	67	
Body Fat Weight		
	74	
Height		

Strategy for Fitness™

Victor L. Vogel

Total Fitness Support Agreement

Attaining total fitness requires the commitment to a healthy nutritional program and workout regimen consistently. Since no one lives in a vacuum, others have an impact on a person's ability to reach total fitness. Spouses, family members, co-workers, customers, and others have to help a person reach their total fitness goal. Realizing this, this agreement is made between [your name] and all those who sign below.

1. I will offer healthy food or other choices during meals, parties, or eating out events.
2. I will refrain from offering unhealthy foods around the house or office.
3. I will provide encouragement to resist unhealthy foods.
4. I will eat healthy foods in front of [you name].
5. When providing food for entertainment, e.g. parties, barbeques, or special events, I will a selection of nourishing and healthy foods when [your name] is attending.
6. I will encourage [your name] to continue to eat correctly and work out consistently.
7. When seeing [your name] with unhealthy food, I will exhort them to resist food temptations.
8. I will provide the personal trainer with honest and accurate information when asked.
9. When around [your name].I will continue to consistently monitor my food, and be conscious about how it could affect [your name].

I enter into this agreement openly and willingly to help [your name] achieve their goal of total fitness. By signing below I represent I will make a good faith effort to honor this agreement at all times.

[Supporter Names]

[Your name]

Date:

Further Fitness Reference Sources

1. www.strategyforfitness.com : Strategy for Fitness™ is a private personal training company focused on private personal training.

2. www.beachbody.com : Provides exercise videos and equipment.

3. www.fitday.com : Is a site that tracks nutrition and exercise. It provides a means for logging food and exercise. The program provides graphs and charts for tracking calories, carbohydrates, fats, and protein as a percent of total calories.

4. www.naturalhealthyellowpages.com : Provides a survey for determining metabolic type. This site provides information for regulating meals to ensure proper use of carbohydrates, proteins, and fats.

5. www.staleytraining.com : Charles Staley runs Staleytraining Systems an organization dedicated to fitness training with an emphasis towards training athletes. This site provides excellent articles on fitness training with a unique approach.

6. www.TheDietSolutionProgram.com : Isabel Del Los Rios provides excellent nutritional information on this web site. She provides free information and has an excellent book "The Diet Solution Program" on nutrition.

7. www.flattenyourabs.net: David Grisaffi's web site provides excellent information on how to exercise effectively, and focuses on abdominal development. David is a highly qualified Kinesiologist and a graduate of the Paul Chek academy. This site provides excellent fitness advice.

8. www.lowglycemicdiet.com : The Fifty50 web site offers information on low glycemic diets and the glycemic index. It also provides a variety of information on how to manage low glycemic meals along with recipes.

9. www.personaltrainertoday.com : The National Federation of Personal Trainers provides electronic articles that provide

information on how to train effectively. The Journal provides access to archived articles ranging from nutrition to exercise.

10. www.nfpt.com : This site is the official personal training certification site for the National Federation of Personal Trainers.

11. www.ez-calculators.com/measurement-conversion-calculator.htm : Provides a tool for converting measurements from metric to English measurements. It also will convert dry and liquid measurements between measurement types, e.g. tablespoon to ounces.

12. www.today.msnbc.msn.com/id/3041426 : This is Today Show's health site. It provides a variety of articles and videos on nutrition, fitness, and health.